HOL[...]
W[...]
MY WEIGHT

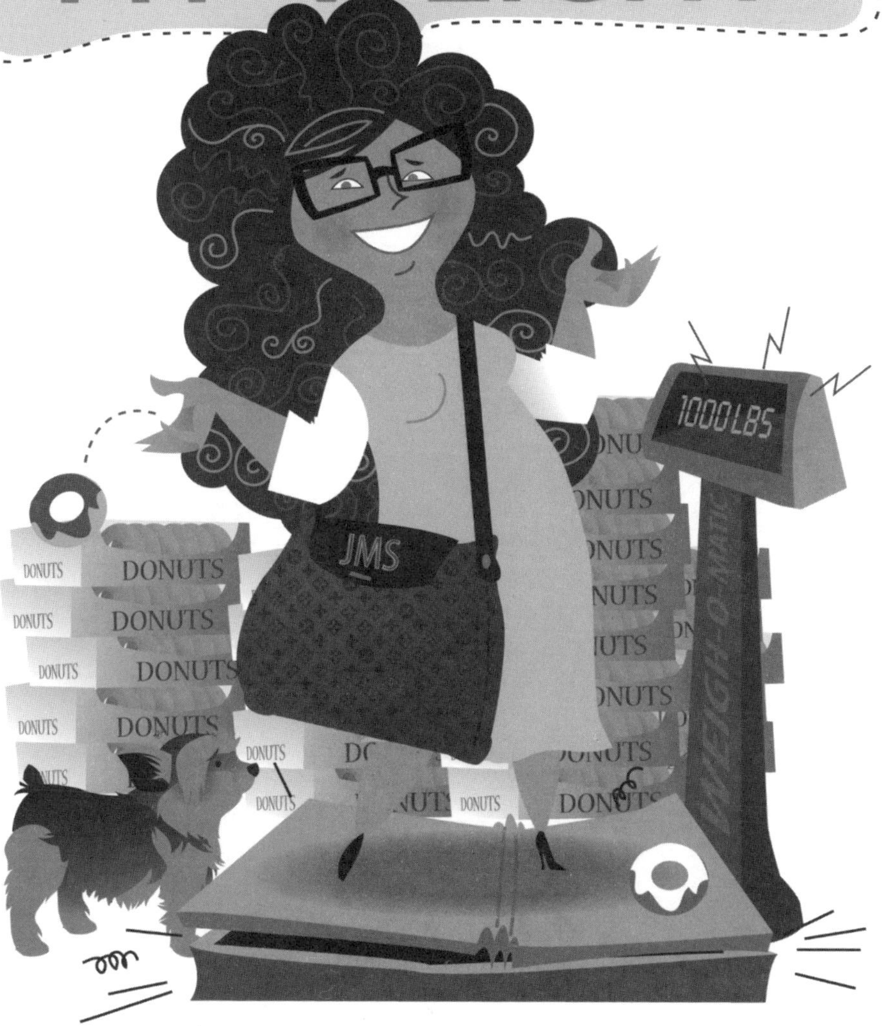

HOLD MY DONUT WHILE I CHECK MY WEIGHT

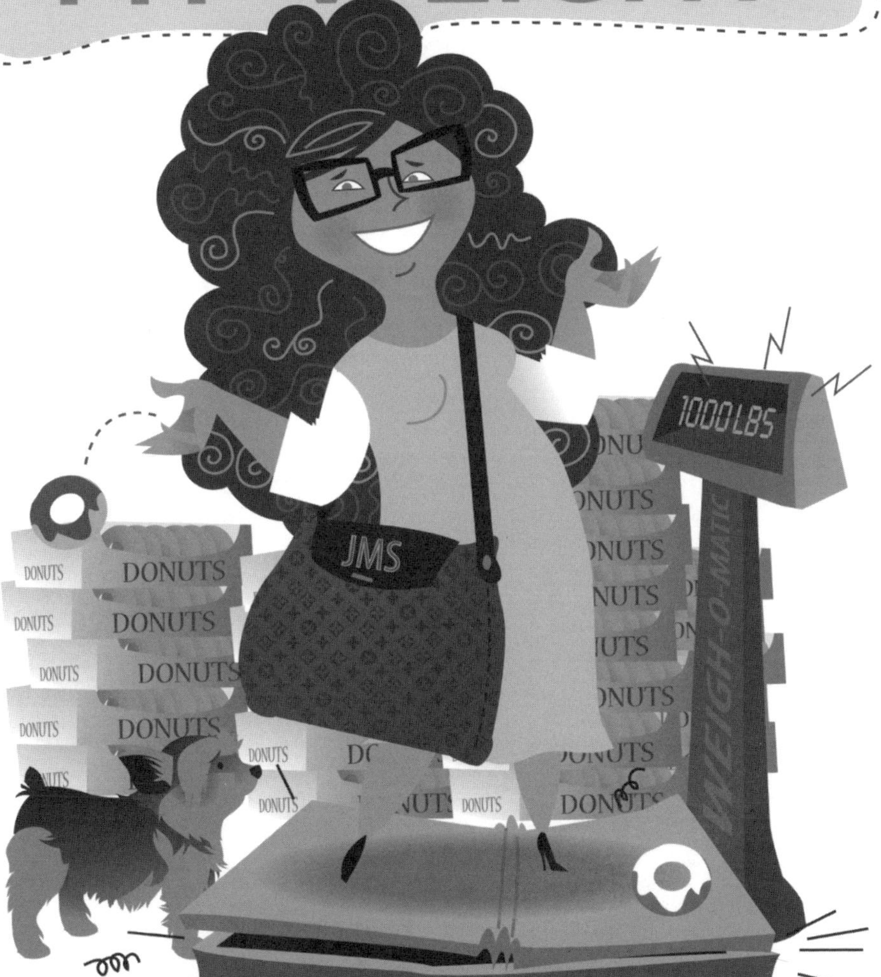

JUDY SHIRLEY

Hold My Donut While I Check My Weight

by Judy Shirley

Hazelwood, MO 63042

All Scripture quotations in this book are from the King James Version of the Bible unless otherwise identified.

Printed in United States of America

WORD AFLAME PRESS
8855 Dunn Road, Hazelwood, MO 63042
www.pentecostalpublishing.com

Library of Congress Cataloging-in-Publication Data

Shirley, Judy.
Hold my donut while I check my weight : when your Kleenex box is empty / by Judy Shirley.
p. cm.
ISBN 978-1-56722-712-3
1. Women—Religious life. 2. Spirituality. 3. Christian life. 4. Weight loss—Religious aspects—Christianity. I. Title.
BV4527.S433 2007
248.8'43—dc22 2007015325

CONTENTS

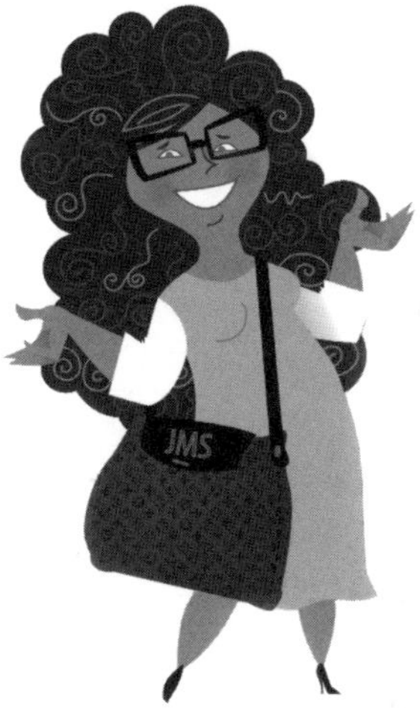

ABOUT THE AUTHOR

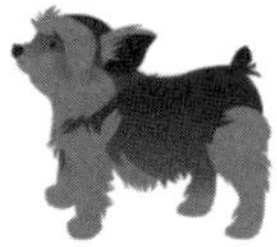

Welcome to the world of the Shirleys, where laughter is an applied medicine. I sincerely hope that you enjoy the comical moments that are supplied in this "dream come true."

Every day I face life as an adventure, never knowing what the outcome will be. It has been my experience that when I've depleted all methods of stress level control, I simply give over to laughter. The Bible states, "The joy of the LORD is [my] strength"! This form of strength-building exercise is the only possible answer to my life.

My life consists of a husband who at times endures me, two very handsome sons who tolerate me, three daughters-in-law who are beautiful, two exceptional grandchildren, and a Yorkshire terrier that allows us to live with her in the home we are paying for! This is the cast of characters that make up my daily activities that cause me to say, "Why did I say that?" These adventures led me to try to make others laugh. A story is always better when you can laugh at yourself, and, believe me, the joke is usually on me.

A host of friends and family, including my parents and siblings, have awaited this expression of comedy that has developed over these many years. My pastor and his lovely wife have given a continual push to this adventure, believing that there is talent for the Lord and

His mighty works hidden in this laughter. To my friends, Kim Johnson and Anita Whittington, a special "thank you" for believing that it would really work out.

A special "thank you" to all at the Pentecostal Publishing House who made this effort of laughter a glorious trail of tears! You enhanced my prayer life.

I sincerely wish the abundance of blessings to each and every one who finds the time to read this material. May God give you laughter and an abundance of it!

Blessings to all,

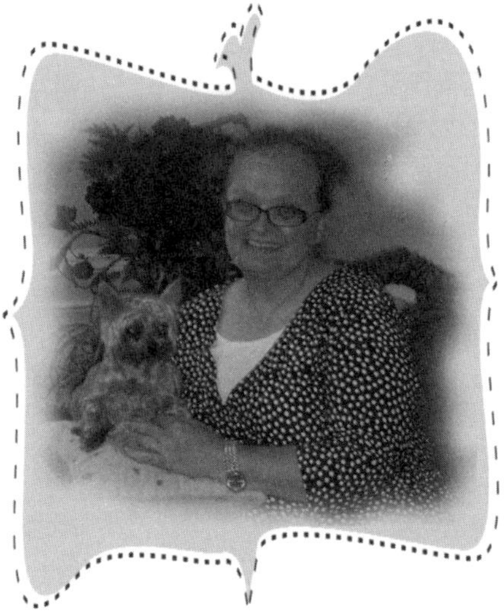

Judy Shirley and
Penny

CHAPTER 1

HOLDING MY DONUT

Donuts, the very epitome of "yum." And yum, unfortunately, is one of my favorite things of life. Yum comes in so many forms, but at this point in my life, yum is represented by my love of donuts.

Not long ago in our area, Krispy Kreme arrived. The pomp and circumstance were unreal. Cars with overweight people in them just waiting to hold those warm, light, delicious donuts in their hands formed lines. The customers digested as many as a dozen at a time, almost a ritual of sorts, trying to see who could hold the most donuts. In fact, some people whom I personally know would get out of bed and drive to Krispy Kreme during the late hours of night just to ingest the calories provided by these donuts. Like me, those folks need the rest more than they need the donuts.

Calories are not your friend. At my age, they are a definite enemy. This enemy tends to control me on levels far beyond my recognition. You know what I mean. There are times when I don't even remember eating the entire dozen donuts. I know you are thinking, "I can't believe she could eat a dozen donuts!" Sure you can. In fact, if I were to go out on a really strong, healthy, close to the ground limb, I would venture to say that the very person holding this book has also held her share of donuts in her hand and in her mouth while complaining about her weight at the same time.

If you eat a cake that has a pound of each ingredient in it, how can that cake not cause you to gain weight? If problems of life weigh on your heart and mind, how can they not take away from the blessings that God is just "waiting" to pour on you?

This reminds me that I do most of my complaining with my mouth full of food. I tend to complain constantly that I can't seem to lose weight. They say appearances count. If true, then I do not need to be eating a dozen donuts when I'm complaining about being overweight. Psalm 25:5 says, "Lead me in thy truth, and teach me: for thou art the God of my salvation; on thee do I wait all day."

The truth of the matter is that sweets are a problem for me, a problem that I can hold in my hand. I am asking God to remove this problem from my taste buds. To avoid these and other sins of the land, I ask that God continually lead me in the truth. He is my only salvation. Not donuts! Not the problems that life present me. The problems of life that I hold so tightly in my clenched fist will also cause my heart to harden.

We, as fine Christians (what other kind is there?), try to appease our situations the same way. We complain to the Lord about our problems while we have a mouth full of the problem, chewing it in small pieces, digesting it to increase our trouble of being overweight. I came to the conclusion that the biggest portion of our overweight problems is from the calories represented in the problems. If donuts are your calorie problem, like they are mine, then the answer is simply, don't eat them. Don't go to the donut shop and ask for a "low-calorie, sugar-free, diet-plan donut." That's not the nature of the donut.

Oh, and for those of you who say, "Well, if you eat them in a sensible manner, you won't have a problem." Right! Define the term "sensible manner." Does that come after the fifth or sixth donut? Here's my favorite terminology, "Let me just have two dozen of those donut holes; that way I'm not consuming as much as a whole donut." Sure thing. Don't forget the Diet Coke that goes with this. After all, watching your weight can be a very trying time. You are trying to find the logic of eating high-calorie foods in order to feed that ever present hunger of stress and the proverbial "I can handle this without the Lord" syndrome. Guess what, folks? The calories are the same in donut holes as those in the big guys. Just because they're smaller doesn't make them diet food. Oh, no! The smaller they are, the easier they pop in your mouth.

So, "Here, hold my donut while I step on the scale!"

CHAPTER 2

STICKY FINGERS

How many times in my life have I struggled with a problem while I was holding it in my hand, refusing to let it go because of sheer and simple control? So many of you are the same. Okay, you may not be overweight, but you struggle every day with a "wait" problem. Sure you do. The weight of our body is the very issue that gives us the understanding to "wait" upon the Lord.

Do I like it or agree with it? No, I don't. But I do have the inner knowledge to know that if the weight on the outside is because of the wait on the inside, then we do have a weight problem.

This is exactly where the donuts arrive in my life. They are simple goodies that, unfortunately, are made hand size. Which, again, fits nicely in your mouth. Isn't it amazing that all the bad calories of food items seem to fit exactly in your mouth? Take broccoli; it's in no way mouth size. That's a good thing. I have nothing against broccoli; it just doesn't fit in my hand like a donut. It doesn't smell as appetizing as a donut, and no matter how many times I wake up during the night, it's never for a craving of broccoli. I have never awakened my husband in the middle of the night to jump in the car and make a mad dash of sixty miles to Krispy Kreme for broccoli spears. They just aren't appealing. But even when gas was my entire paycheck, those donuts would call. The miles were a mere misfortune of life. However, if you think about it, those wee morning-hour cravings save on gas. No traffic. Just a quick breeze to the other side of town. Then again, so are the state troopers. They do have twenty-four-hour shifts that, I might add, are usually donut equipped. When you do arrive at the donut shop in those wee hours of morning, if you happen to be behind a police officer in any form of unmarked car, don't honk your horn, flash your lights, or scream uncontrollable donut obscenities as you wait in line. Donuts are cheaper by the dozen without the benefit of a traffic ticket.

Problems. Like donuts, they come in all sizes and shapes. Whether I'm aware of them or not, I tend to hold problems as I do donuts, firmly and with admiration. You ask, how can you admire problems? We do it every day. How do I know? Because we won't let go of them. We hold them snugly in our hands and "admire" them all day long. This admiration is not unlike the way I handle donuts. I'm worried about being overweight, so I have a donut to help me cope with my worry. Problems always weigh more than they should. And, as intelligent as we humans are, we tend to add weight to an already overweight problem.

I use myself for an example because at one time in my life—a million years ago—I was smaller in physical size. Over the course of my life both my consumption of food and my inclination to completely control my problems have expanded. However, the need to control my problems has backfired. I should have turned them over to the Lord. He doesn't have a weight problem. Have you read anywhere in the Bible the words "diet," "sugar-free," or "stress controlled"? They aren't there. You don't even have to look. Take my word for it. When God tells us to lay our problems at His feet, it's a form of biblical Weight Watchers. You will lose a tremendous amount of burden (worry weight) when you lay them at Jesus' feet. Do we do it? No, we tend to run to Jesus, describe and complain about our problem, lay it at His feet, turn around, and pick it up ever so quickly. Now, where are the problems? You guessed it; you're holding them in your hand, and you're admiring them.

So, "Here, hold my donut while I step on the scale!"

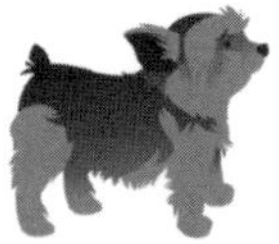

CHAPTER 3

SUGAR-COATED MEMORIES

When I was growing up, at least a hundred years ago, it was a very special treat to have donuts from Shipley Donuts. At that time, Shipley was the only donut shop in town. My three brothers and I would devour those donuts. My favorite was always the long johns. You know the ones, long pastries filled with enough white sugary crème to sink a large cruise ship and drizzled chocolate on top. At that time I could eat several and never know it. Who knew that it would take forty years for those donuts to poof out? I am living proof that combustion of donuts takes forty years, and then they explode, all over your body.

Combustible donuts—wouldn't that be an advertising phrase? How many people would buy donuts or pastries if the advertising description was not appealing? However, if I start to describe the smell of a fresh donut, your mouth begins to water for one. If your town does not have a donut shop, the grocery store carries the little pre-boxed donuts, the ones with all the white sugar on the outside. Do they taste like a donut? Sure they do, especially when you are craving a donut. Do problems seem like problems when you hold on to them? Sure they do. But just like the pre-boxed donuts, we package them differently. We call them "stress"!

Isn't "stress" a wonderful word? Actually, the Christian meaning of this word should be "prayer life." If you have a prayer life, your stress level is lower. God will completely take care of all problems. Now, does He give the same answer to problems as we do? No! And that is a good thing. He is the author of life. He knows all. We are . . . nothing. Look, if He can start with nothing and create the world, including us—and remember we are nothing compared to the wonders of heaven—then why in the world do we package our problems as pre-boxed donuts? We accept an inferior form of a donut when what we really want is the donut shop donuts across town. But because of convenience and the "I'm in control" issue, we consume those pre-boxed donuts and complain about our weight. Stress adds weight. This falls under the "problems are full of calories" law. Haven't heard of that law? You have now. The longer you hold on to a problem, the more it weighs. I don't know about you, but in my case if I continue to add calories to my already over-caloried problem, my stress level will have to be renamed. It will then become a full-fledged breakdown, one of such magnitude that I will then have to depend on God to bring it under control.

So, "Here, hold my donut while I step on the scale!"

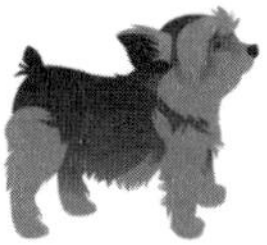

CHAPTER 4

WHAT KIND OF DONUT AM I HOLDING?

I once told someone at work that everything on me hurt. The real problem is, I can't find everything. It's hidden between the combustible donuts and those absolutely scrumptious double cheeseburgers that I ate when I was eighteen years old. Sometimes I think it would be better if we started life as senior citizens and gained our youth as we live. In other words, if I knew in my first-grade class what I know now, I could have flown through school instead of worrying about recess. Recess is that time when you get to run, jump, scream, and eat snacks. Those snacks that we thought we ran off in recess are now present in pounds. A good phrase for those would be "recessed pounds." That sounds good, doesn't it? Recessed usually means hidden away or something. Here again, I have the "or something."

It's always the "or somethings" in life that drive us to the donut shops. The "or somethings" tend to overwhelm us beyond our ability to understand. You have said it as many times as I have: "I don't understand why this is happening to me. I'm doing everything I know to do to serve God!" Good for you. Continue in that phase of life. If everything you know to do is within His commandments, then you are on the right road. If your "controlling" issue is taking over, then beware. Donut shops are not a Weight Watchers' meeting. You don't meet people there who are having extreme weight problems that demand a prescription of dozens of donuts for weight control. It just doesn't happen. I wish it did, but it isn't logical. If you're allergic to chocolate, why would you continue to eat candy bars? Just to see how fast you can get to the hospital? I don't think so. People, myself included, who are in the overweight phase of life are always trying to separate the good from the bad. Sounds like a Christian's guidebook. I believe that would be the Bible. The good from the bad. I often think of those rice cakes I purchase every once in a while. I laughingly describe them as "cardboard sandwiches." They crunch like cardboard does. And just think, you and I actually pay good gas money to purchase those cakes. We then eat them and drink a Diet Coke along with them. Are we for real or what?

It is this series of "or somethings" that brings me to appreciate the irony that sometimes comes with life. Why am I overweight? If I am blessed to have "happy" birthdays then I am blessed to have a changing body style. Sounds like an automobile maker, doesn't it? Much like automobiles, every year our bodies tend to change. As life blesses us we move from economy models to the luxury car. These cars are larger and more impressive. Obviously we don't mind because it doesn't stop us from waiting in line at the donut shop.

So, "Here, hold my donut while I step on the scale!"

CHAPTER 5

SUGAR-FREE DONUTS

Donuts are an ever-present problem for me. First of all, when they are fresh out of the oven, the aroma is impossible to resist. The smell operates like a camouflage outfit. Calories hide behind the smell, much like the devil. At times, he is hidden in what appears to be a harmless situation. The donut aroma meets with my nose, and my inner self knows it's a donut that I smell. Do we always know it's the devil that attracts us? No, we don't. Just like the donut, it's only after I inhale that delightful smell and indulge in the calories do I begin to think about the results of my choice. So it is with the devil. Many times it's after that fact that we realize the results of the choices we have made. Are donuts a good choice? If you're able to handle the calories that are hidden between the layers of pastry and sugar they are, but I can't.

I am warned by an inner conscience that says, "Wait. This is not what you need!" Does it upset me? Yes, it does. Because, as you have been made aware, I love donuts.

This love of donuts, associated with other loves of life, has had an outstanding effect on my life. Don't think for one instant that because you are dealing with an overweight problem, you can't work for God. Poof on that one! That's a trick of the skinny demons. Let me tell you this: for years, and I do mean years, I have desired to be a writer. Isn't that pretty funny? In actuality, I have written stuff all my life. My mother had this same desire. Her life ended at a very young age that left her desire unfulfilled, except vicariously through me. Here I am. I may not be a well-known author by any means, but when God gives the words that appear on paper for others to read and associate with their lives, that places me in His will and the problem is solved. God's benefits are outstanding. Most companies offer a 401k plan today instead of a retirement program. God offers an eternity of gold under your feet. How enchanting! The very precious metal here on earth is but a stepping-stone in heaven.

Present-day problems are an everyday happening. I am aware that people handle situations differently. For this, I offer a heartfelt prayer to those who can't handle issues in their life. Mine tend to lead me to laughter. It's amazing to hear someone laugh. Even when tears are in my eyes, someone laughing will bring a smile to my face. The "or somethings" in life drain us of laughter. Laughter is a good medicine for almost any situation. It will allow the combustible part of those donuts you inhaled to vanish. Of course, a good long walk wouldn't hurt either. Look at ways to keep yourself busy, whether in the house or out. As mentioned, walk off the calories of the donuts. Walk off the worry of the problem. I can't say that I truly do this on a consistent basis, but I want to. The desire is there. The next step to the problem is . . . the next step.

So, "Here, hold my donut while I step on the scale!"

CHAPTER 6

ALL KINDS OF DONUTS

Donuts aren't the only food I really love. I have the same affection toward other things. For instance, blackberry cobbler was made in heaven. No other place could have created such a wonder of life. Peaches—just the mention makes me smile. These special flavors of life are what hold my weight in place. I love them. Every day I have to ask the Lord to help me not eat every candy bar in the vending machine. While I would never do this, simply because I can't afford the inflated cost of the candy in the vending machine, the urge is a constant in my life. You'll notice that I didn't say that I wouldn't try to eat all the candy bars in the vending machine, only that I couldn't afford to.

Can I afford to "wait" on the Lord to take complete control? I must learn to. It's a constant battle illustrated by my prayer "Here, Lord, let me hold the problem until I know you have the answer in my other hand." Do you think He holds back the good stuff until we allow Him to give it to us? I wonder about that. I am so guilty of holding on. Again, remember I said, "The results of your choices." It's my choice to hold on to my problem, not God's! He is ever present and willing to take full and complete control of all problems *if* I let go. I can't. Why not? Because of the "wait" problem. You guessed it. I am unable to wait on the Lord, so I appease myself with the flavors that help to give me control: Donuts, blackberry cobbler, peaches.

There are so many good things to eat in this life. I try not to take anything for granted. Enjoy that wonderful five-dollar cup of coffee. Can you believe we pay more for a cup of coffee than we do for a gallon of milk? Or, for that matter, a gallon of gas? But we do so because we like the coffee. It's only expensive when we don't need it. That's our motto.

So, "Here, hold my donut while I step on the scale!"

CHAPTER 7

THE "WAIT" ASSOCIATED WITH THE DONUT

My pastor taught a lesson recently about the woman at the well and the twelve disciples who went into town and bypassed their blessing on the way. Why? Because they had a "flavor" on their mind. They were too busy holding their problem in their hand to realize the blessing right next to them. Jesus, on the other hand, never saw the problem. He simply saw the blessing. The woman at the well, much like me, tried to control her "wait" problem. She waited until there was no one around before she filled her water pitcher. But she never expected that someone was "waiting" on her.

Who is standing next to you at Wal-Mart? Do you know? Did you know that people are desperate for someone to talk to? A simple "hello" can be the beginning of a treasured friendship. A good listening ear—and mind you, not a gossiping tongue—is invaluable. Just because you hear it doesn't mean you have to tell it. When I was growing up that was called a "tattletale"! Don't be one. My dad always used to say, "Secrets are like pie crusts, easily broken!" He's right. So if you know a secret and just have to tell it, tell Jesus. He's your safest bet. Besides that, He already knows it, as well as a lot more that you have no idea about. He sees inside and out. So He sees you holding that donut and gulping down those sodas. He knows, whether your weight coach does or not. He also knows how long your "wait" has been bothering you. Remember, His time is not our time. That's a good thing because I never have enough time. And the time I do have I often use very foolishly.

So, "Hold my donut while I step on the scale."

CHAPTER 8

WHICH DONUT SATISFIES YOUR SWEET TOOTH?

Donuts and weight. They go together. If you pick one, the other will greet you in the mirror not many days hence. Wait and Jesus. They go together. If you pick one, the other will greet you every moment of the day for as long as you will accept and love Him.

As I hold on to my donut, I tend to check my weight every few hours, just to see if I've lost anything. As long as the donut is in my hand it represents the fact that I can control the problem. When I lay the problem at Jesus' feet and walk away, I no longer worry about the "wait."

My journey continues. Is it the donut or the weight? Which one do I choose today? Without fail, I'm back to the most antagonizing question I know. The very solution that I have chosen to solve my problem—the one I'm holding in my hand—is the very problem I will face at another turn of life. My love of donuts causes the problem of snug-fitting clothes. I solve that by purchasing new clothes. Then I tend to eat again because I'm disgusted with the larger size clothes. It's the vicious circle of my life. Whether I chose to agree or disagree, the end result is the same whether I am in control, or think I'm in control. Wrong! Whether my preference is to hold the donut in my left hand or my other hand, neither hand is right!

Is it the weight or the wait that I am having the most trouble with? To tell the truth, it's the "wait." But the "wait" holds the most blessed assurance. Jesus is always there. He understands. What I fail to realize is that God has no problem with "wait." His time is not ours. Therefore, He never has to wait! His promise to never leave us nor forsake us should be all the "wait" insurance we need. It's this constant battle inside myself that detours me from the feet of Jesus and back to my donut.

There is absolutely no doubt in my mind that God is the answer to all my problems. In fact, I testify to others that without Him, I cannot breathe the next breath of life that He so graciously gives me. If I could put as much trust in Him as I do a box of donuts, I would be an unstoppable Christian. My "wait" with God is determined by my desire, just like my "weight" is determined by donuts.

Does He understand our weight problem? Yes, but He isn't going to help us when we decide to eat the whole dozen of donuts. However, the problem we have in our right hand is never right. It's when we put it in His hand that our weight changes. "Wait" is one of the hardest words spoken by parents, teachers, or innocent bystanders. "Wait"—the hardest secret to any success. "Wait"—the hardest moments to watch as the hands of the clock turn. "Wait"—the most loving words God can share with us. Why? Because "But they that wait upon the LORD shall renew their strength; they shall mount up with wings as eagles; they shall run, and not be weary; and they shall walk, and not faint" (Isaiah 40:31). See, even without the donuts, the Lord promises you will not faint.

Donuts—or the problems that we face each day—whether job loss, financial worries, family problems, or inner self problems, are all controlled by putting our complete trust in God. Although this is easy to say it is one of the hardest things I have found to do. Why? Because, like most people, I tend to want to control and schedule everything in my life and my family's lives. I take this very human trait to Jesus every day. And, every day He presents Himself as the creator and miracle worker of my life.

Donuts are life's way of weighing me down. The problems I insist upon carrying alone are the devil's way of causing confusion and distraction to my recognition of God's ever-present presence. God is not the author of confusion. So when I become confused about what problem I am holding or why I'm holding it, I have to quickly realize that the enemy has propelled into my life and is stealing the answer right before my eyes. The desire of the enemy is to pull me away from God through depression. This is a common occurrence in our lives that often comes from the added pressure that we place upon ourselves. We try to be what everyone else expects us to be, not what God has placed in our hearts to be. We can solve this simple problem by praising His name for the victory that is at hand.

The problems of my life have not subsided. The human side of me says they will continue to cause havoc whenever possible in a physical way. However, I am not reaching for the donuts as often as I did. My spiritual side has assured me through the many prayers of others and my increasing prayer life that "all is well with my soul." The desire of my heart is to serve God and allow Him to give my soul the peace that comes from being under His control. What a wonderful blessing He has promised, a gift that I long to be able to share with others! It will allow me to experience and to share an eternal answer to an earthly problem.

Whether the problems of life are glazed, plain, or sugar coated, they still are problems. When laid at His feet they become opportunities for miracles—miracles that have been promised to us as we walk by faith and not by sight. Sometimes we fail to see these miracles as we "wait" upon the Master's guiding hand. Our loving God has already carried the "weight" of the world upon His heart, causing us to be free of the "weight" of sin in our lives.

May God bless you. May you live long in His precious Holy Spirit and prosper. And may your "wait" be only a small problem in your life.

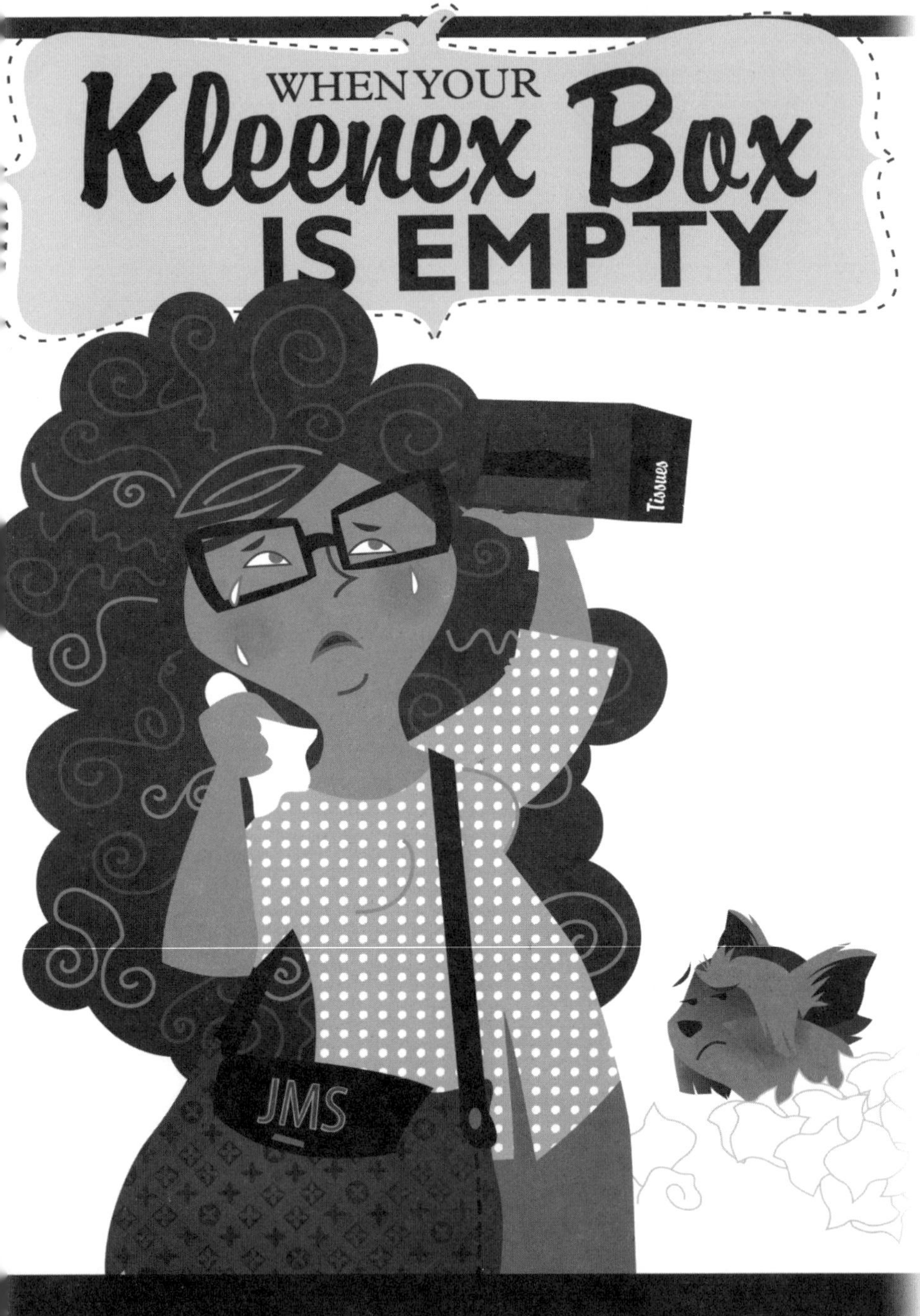
WHEN YOUR
Kleenex Box
IS EMPTY
Tissues
JMS

WHEN YOUR Kleenex Box IS EMPTY

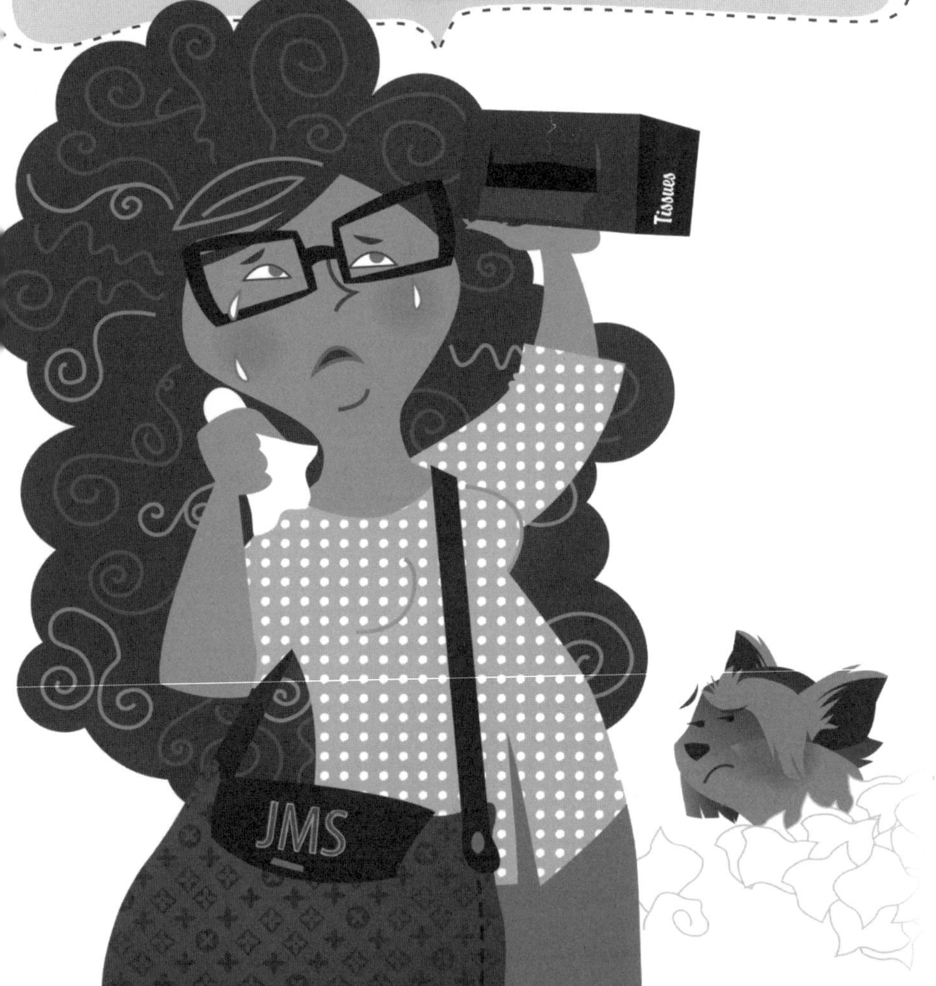

JUDY SHIRLEY

When Your Kleenex Box Is Empty

by Judy Shirley

Hazelwood, MO 63042

All Scripture quotations in this book are from the King James Version of the Bible unless otherwise identified.

Printed in United States of America

WORD AFLAME PRESS
8855 Dunn Road, Hazelwood, MO 63042
www.pentecostalpublishing.com

Library of Congress Cataloging-in-Publication Data

Shirley, Judy.
Hold my donut while I check my weight : when your Kleenex box is empty / by Judy Shirley.
p. cm.
ISBN 978-1-56722-712-3
1. Women—Religious life. 2. Spirituality. 3. Christian life. 4. Weight loss—Religious aspects—Christianity. I. Title.
BV4527.S433 2007
248.8'43—dc22 2007015325

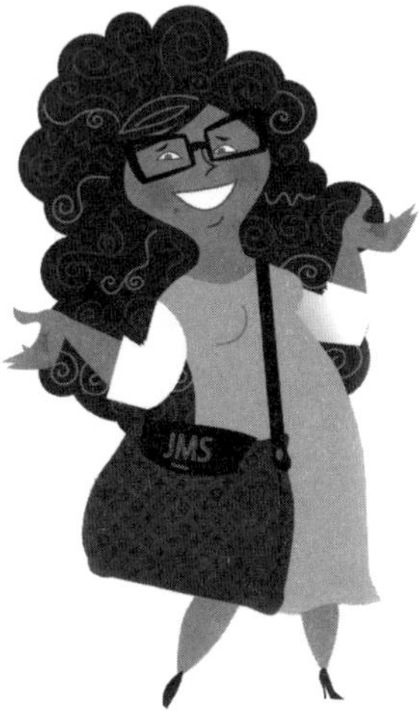

ABOUT THE AUTHOR

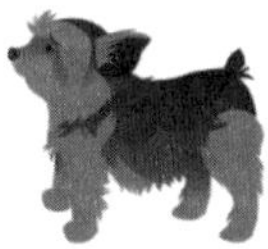

Welcome to the world of the Shirleys, where laughter is an applied medicine. I sincerely hope that you enjoy the comical moments that are supplied in this "dream come true."

Every day I face life as an adventure, never knowing what the outcome will be. It has been my experience that when I've depleted all methods of stress level control, I simply give over to laughter. The Bible states, "The joy of the LORD is [my] strength"! This form of strength-building exercise is the only possible answer to my life.

My life consists of a husband who at times endures me, two very handsome sons who tolerate me, three daughters-in-law who are beautiful, two exceptional grandchildren, and a Yorkshire terrier that allows us to live with her in the home we are paying for! This is the cast of characters that make up my daily activities that cause me to say, "Why did I say that?" These adventures led me to try to make others laugh. A story is always better when you can laugh at yourself, and, believe me, the joke is usually on me.

A host of friends and family, including my parents and siblings, have awaited this expression of comedy that has developed over these many years. My pastor and his lovely wife have given a continual push to this adventure, believing that there is talent for the Lord and

His mighty works hidden in this laughter. To my friends, Kim Johnson and Anita Whittington, a special "thank you" for believing that it would really work out.

A special "thank you" to all at the Pentecostal Publishing House who made this effort of laughter a glorious trail of tears! You enhanced my prayer life.

I sincerely wish the abundance of blessings to each and every one who finds the time to read this material. May God give you laughter and an abundance of it!

Blessings to all,

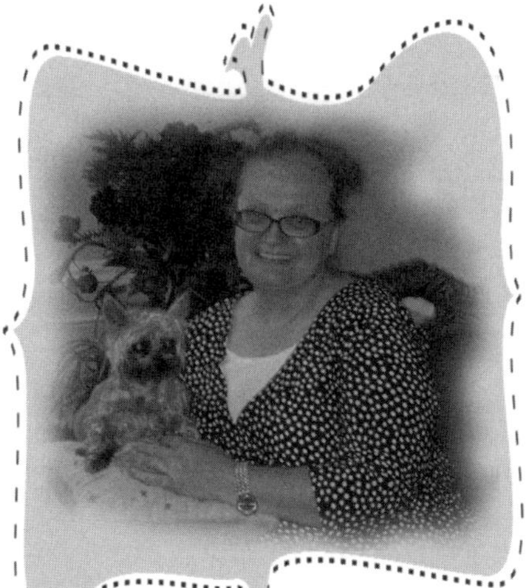

Judy Shirley and
Penny

WHEN YOUR Kleenex Box IS EMPTY

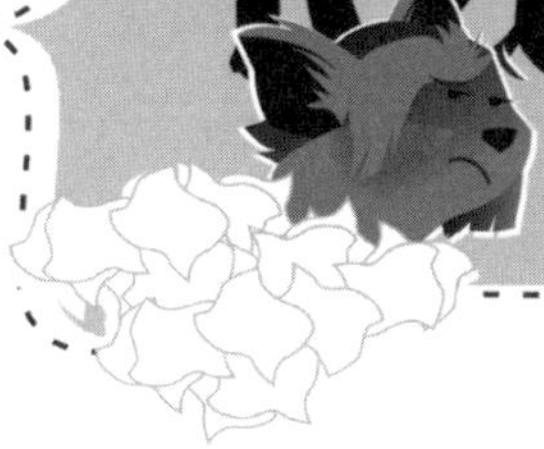

How many boxes of Kleenex do you have in your home at this given moment? Depending on the season, this count could be more than you think. Kleenex is as much a part of our home as the paper towels in the kitchen. In fact, sometimes the paper towels are my Kleenex. They are the survival items of nature. Kleenex, paper towels, and toilet paper—don't leave home without them. If you still have small children in your world, add a container of wipes to this basic survivor's kit. Just when you think you've outgrown the need of wipes, you spill coffee or cola on your clothes on your way to work. And this is the day you are interviewing for the promotion you've worked for over the past five years. Yes, now is when the $6.99 stain-resistant wipes look like a great bargain. That and the turbo engine in your car! You can always rush in and wash out the stain before your interview. So instead of a simple stain, you will now sport a large wet spot that is more easily explained than a mere coffee stain. Right!

If you have children—and most of us do in some form or fashion—whether big or small they still demand a Kleenex every once in a while. They help to keep their noses clean and to catch the tears that fall when they encounter the word "No." Our grown-up children still react in much the same way as the grandchildren who have now arrived on the scene. My grandchildren act better than their mother and father at times.

With my emotions all over the place, it's not unusual for me to cry at the drop of a hat or when the neighbor's cat crosses the street. Either way it's pure and simple drama for me. I've always had a tender spot for certain things—the sun coming up or going down, the size of the moon, if the grass is green or brown. I mean really, I can get up on Saturday morning and be emotional about something before the clock strikes 8 AM. That's because the good Lord made me this way. Or maybe it's the fact that I'm old! When you're of a certain age, you have to cry to relieve some of the water pressure in your hands and feet. Otherwise, you would waddle around with hands and feet larger than normal. You may think I'm trying to pull one over on you, but sometimes I have enough water in my fingers to drown a good three-dollar goldfish. Let's not go to the feet. Swollen, tired, and puffy! Then the doctors give you "water pills" to help with the water. That's a big help, or it would be if I could stay at my desk long enough to get something done. So Kleenex tissues are an ample part of my life. I can't be satisfied with one. My crying spells require much more than that. A handful at a time, and remember this is just Saturday morning.

I can hear something sad on the radio and have to pull to the side of the road to pull myself together. It

takes me thirty minutes to get ready for work, and then my emotions perk up and it takes me fifteen minutes to pull myself back together. It always makes you feel good when you arrive at work and the first comment they say is, "Boy, what happened to you?" I always tell them that I had to work over an hour to look like this.

Emotions—good or bad—belong to us. Different people react differently in similar situations. What may completely destroy you may only be a drop in the hat for me and vice versa. These emotions are just part of the woman that God created. We often label these people as "moody" folks. This is true of most of us. Most of us are not in the mood to do whatever it is we're doing, especially if it is our 8 AM–5 PM job. My pastor spoke recently about working in the church. Is your work for the church a ministry or a job? If you love it and enjoy the pleasure of doing it, it's a ministry. If you seek praise and become prideful, it's a job. It was a very good message. It hit my heart. How can I present God with my talent if I demand praises from others? The demand for praise would make it a job and not the ministry God intended it to be.

Do you become emotional over someone mowing the grass? Maybe you should. I've seen people taking care of their lawns when they could barely maneuver around. Why? Because they love what they are doing! Do you love what you are doing? Most of us would say, "No!" We love it when others know we are doing something! There is a difference. Lord, grant us the ability to love and respond to your spirit of giving. Teach us to give financially and with compassion. After all, just because you are rich in one area doesn't mean you are rich in another. I

have seen people who are blessed with very good paying positions but they are so depressed they cannot go to work. On the flip side, I have talked with people who do not have enough money to pay for their basic needs but they have compassion and are so rich with a radiant love of Jesus that their finances are met through the faith and mercy of kindness. They never worry, nor do they complain. What witness to the fruit of the Spirit! Wouldn't it be wonderful to be able to overlook our own needs in order to inspire those around us with our compassion?

Compassion is not an easy thing for some people because it involves an unselfish spirit—willingness to give until it hurts. However, the closer our walk with God, the easier it is to not be selfish in all things. We, as humans, tend to believe that this is only applicable finances. It is not. I've seen a time when someone would deliver groceries or send a card in the mail, and that would be the turning point of someone else's faith in God. How wonderful to be used of God in this manner! A simple prayer or a testimony of a victorious triumph over a trial is worth more than you know.

I encourage you to take someone under your wing. Help to strengthen their love for the Lord. In doing so, you will be surprised at your ability to grow and nourish your soul. Nothing is more satisfying than spreading as much love as you can to a hungry soul. It's a mutual blessing.

This brings me back to my empty box of Kleenex. Compassion and Kleenex go together. You cannot extend compassion without a humble heart. To be broken with compassion is worth at least a box of tissue. You see, when God breaks our heart, out of that broken spirit will

flow a river (and I do mean a river) of tears. The tears will first wash away all of the built-up residue in our hearts, making way for the compassion for others to take its place. A compassionate heart is worth so much more than any value assigned by an appraiser. So is a box of Kleenex. What do you do when your Kleenex box is empty? Rejoice! Rejoice for the victory that is present. Rejoice for the sheer delight of rejoicing. Rejoice for the person who is going to receive the blessing. Just rejoice and find another box of tissues. You will need them when you see the miracles that provide answers to your prayers.

I've complained so many times to my stepmother over the fact that all I can do is cry when the Lord's Spirit moves on me. She always laughs at me and says the same thing every time, "Tears are a language that God understands!" Tears are a pure language of the heart. They are also humbling. The way to humble your heart before the Lord is to completely and unselfishly open up your entire being to His molding of your soul. This humbling experience requires the use of the Kleenex box again—at times more than one Kleenex box. With the use of those Kleenex comes the second phase that we tend to bypass. Rejoice. Rejoice. Rejoice in praise and rejoice in song. So what if you can't carry a tune in a bucket with the lid attached? Even people who have magnificent voices are taught to sing. Ask God to teach you to sing from the heart. Being in tune with God reaches more souls than being in tune with music. Being in tune with God lasts an eternity. Being in tune with music lasts until the last note of the "sound of the trumpet."

What exactly brings us to the emotional state of

tears? The death of a loved one, finances (as I have stated many times), family problems, job issues (the loss of which I am facing for the second time in my life), friendships, weight problems, health problems—the list will never grow smaller. Here again we are met with the Kleenex box. Your prayer time will also affect the Kleenex box. A one-minute prayer will usually not require a Kleenex. A thirty-minute prayer will. An hour-long prayer will require several Kleenexes. An outstanding praise and worship service at church uses lots of Kleenexes. Judge your Kleenex needs by your prayer life. Oh my! Some of you have the same amount of prayer as you have tissues in your handbag—none! Help us, Lord. Help us to be drawn to your presence for pure and simple praise.

When you pray, do you pray for yourself or others? If your first answer is others, then I would have a hard time believing you. Most of us start our prayer life with "Bless me, Lord." If you don't, then I hope God will bless you with a double portion. If you do, then I still ask God to give you a blessing with a double portion. You see, whether I start my prayer life one way or the other, I feel it is important to recognize the fact that I'm in His presence. No one else offers the love that we need to take care of the empty box of Kleenex.

You see, the empty box of Kleenex simply represents the fact that you have been broken to His touch. Whether it's a simple brush (another wonderful message I heard from Brother Nathan Cannon) or a complete touch, either way, He is in your life. When God touches us, we are never the same—inside or outside! Who wants to be like everyone else? Not me. I want to be just like God wants

me to be. If laughter is what is needed to carry me through a problem, and the ability to share that laughter with others in the same situation is needed, Lord, use me for your purpose. This is a risky prayer, because in order for me to be used of God, I have to go through the trial myself. But knowing that He is guiding me means more than the world to me. As He guides me, He talks to me. He points out areas that need attention. He directs me to others. He directs others to me. He takes it slow and easy so that He is a constant friend, always at my side. He never goes ahead of me and leaves me stranded. He never forgets to speak to me, to let me know He is there, like the shepherd He is. To know His voice and recognize it as He speaks, in itself contributes to Kleenex time. The stillness of His voice can cause the seas to calm, the winds to ease, the storms of our life to settle. Can anyone else offer you this peace and just for the price of a box of Kleenex? No. Not even close.

The rich and powerful look for the easy way out, spending untold amounts of money to find pleasure and comfort for their souls, when all that is needed is a simple box of Kleenex! They cannot afford the price it takes to become humble. That is, until God moves upon their hearts. The rich man cried from across the great gulf, asking that someone be sent to tell his brother to avoid damnation. Do you think at that time in his life he would have cared about the cost of a box of Kleenex? The cost would not have been questioned. Is a second chance at eternity worth a box of Kleenex? It should be. For the rich man, a simple drop of water was his only request. Not much to ask for when everything around you is in flames.

A simple box of Kleenex tissue! Full, it signifies the

opportunity you have to be in His presence. Empty, it provides the assurance of the victory ahead. Lord, how willing am I to look at a box of Kleenex tissues? Do I see the opportunity for myself only, or am I willing to empty my heart for others? Either way, that box of tissue has the drawing power to set me at His feet to receive far greater blessings than my soul can contain. Remember, the next time your problems of life are too much to handle, purchase a box of tissue, talk to God, and your answer will arrive.